The Abdominoplasty

(illustrated)

By
Lynne D M Noble

Copyright 2018 Lynne D M Noble

This book shall not, by way of trade or otherwise, be lent, re-sold, hired out, or otherwise circulated without the prior consent of the copyright holder or the publisher in any form of binding or cover than that in which it is published and without a similar condition including this condition being imposed on the subsequent purchaser.
The use of its contents in another media is also subject to the same conditions.

Independently published

Preface

Mummy tummy is a common condition in those who have had pregnancies but it all occurs in people with connective tissue disorders – both male and female – and for those whose occupations involve heavy lifting. Sometimes there appears to be no cause whatsoever. On other occasions, people combine abdominoplasty with liposuction to deal with areas they are not happy with and which may cause physical or emotional difficulties.

This book looks at the journey of one individual's abdominoplasty and the common complications following surgery.

The Abdominoplasty

Abdominoplasties are not just carried out for cosmetic reasons only. Sometimes they are carried out because a diastasis rectus will have occurred. This is commonly referred to as 'mummy tummy' in which a gap opens up between the abdominal muscles. This leaves the internal organs unprotected.

Normally the gap will be small. However, at a gap of 1.7cm or more, then problems do occur as the internal organs will not be held in their correct places.

Difficulties with back pain are not uncommon. It might be difficult standing up for more than a few minutes. I know of a neighbour who had to lean over the garden gate to support herself if talking to a neighbour.

The separation of muscles can occur anywhere in the midline or all the way down. The abdominal muscles are connected by a thin tissue called the linea alba.

Any pressure within the abdominal cavity has the potential to cause these muscles to spread. In some cases, the connective tissue may also split.

This is more likely to occur with those with connective tissue disorders such as Ehlers Danlos Syndrome. However, pregnancy is by far the most likely cause of diastasis recti which is why the condition is referred to a mummy tummy.

There are a range of exercises which are supposed if the separation doesn't go back after pregnancy, after a reasonable time. However, I do not know of anyone for whom these have worked.

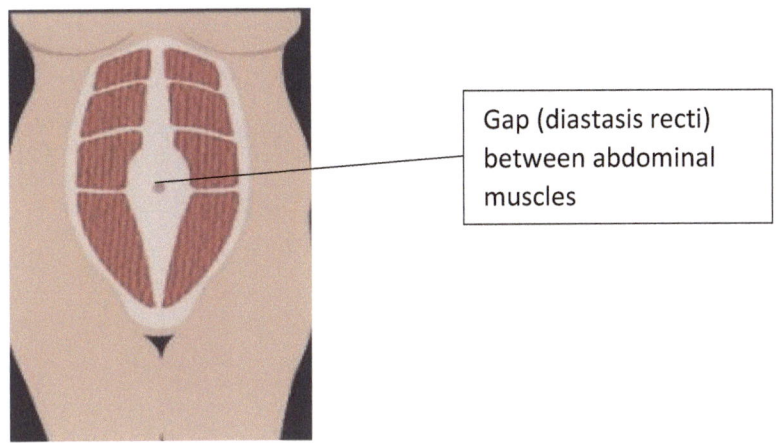

Gap (diastasis recti) between abdominal muscles

My diastasis was not a mere 1.7cm or less. The abdominal separation that I had was 12cm which is a very large rift.

In spite of numerous trips to the GP regarding this huge bump that I had, no one thought to tell me that it was a diastasis and a wide one at that.

It was only when I approached a plastic surgeon that I was at last given a name for the bump. This was after I had wasted hundreds of pounds on treatment for lymphoedema, thinking it was that (the practitioner didn't tell me otherwise since she was raking in my money) and spent years not being to find clothes which fitted over this bump.

I had been unable to stand up for more than a few minutes and had persistent backache.

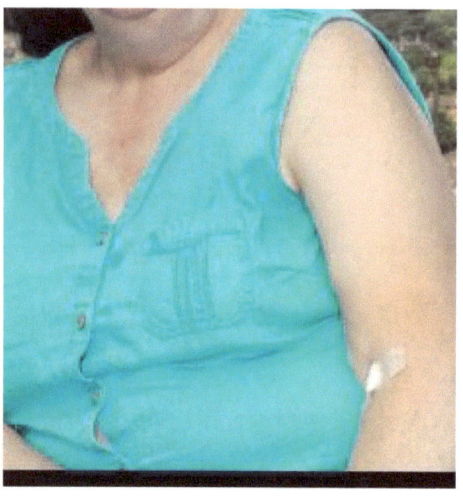

The 'bulge' at the midriff is not fat. It is due to the abdominal separation.

The Operation

The operation was scheduled for the 13th September and I had a number of pre-operative blood tests to check that I was in a healthy state.

Due to the size of the abdominal gap I was informed that the operation would take six hours but, in reality, it took nine hours.

I wasn't really bothered how long it would take. I just wanted to wear some decent clothes!

The surgeon had explained that they would have to make a hip to hip cut before flipping the skin back and pulling the muscles back to where they should be. Then he would use four layers of sutures to keep it in place forever.

Before I went to the operating theatre, the consultant drew on me to show which bits he was going to correct.

Of course, I have no recollection of the actual operation. When I awoke I was informed that there had been complications.

Apparently, I have very thin veins. These broke up as soon as the anaesthetist put the needle in. A couple of days when all the bruising came out, my arms and hands were covered. The picture below is the first area where the anaesthetist tried to obtain a good vein. The bruising did get worse than this.

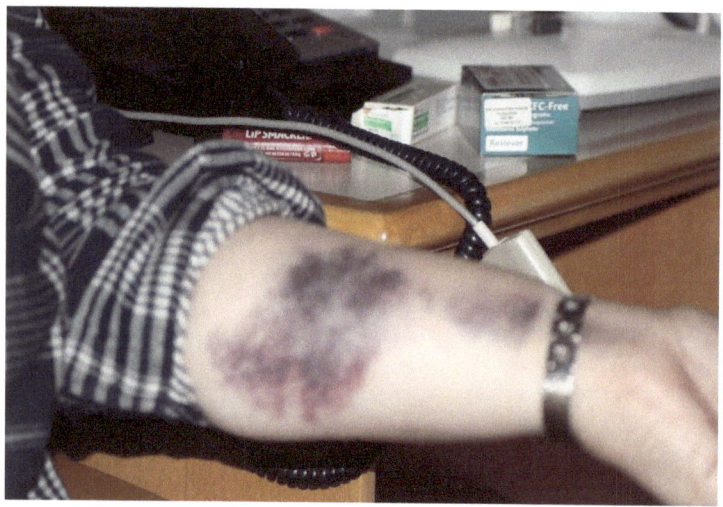

But, as you can see below, the bulge where the diastasis had been had gone.

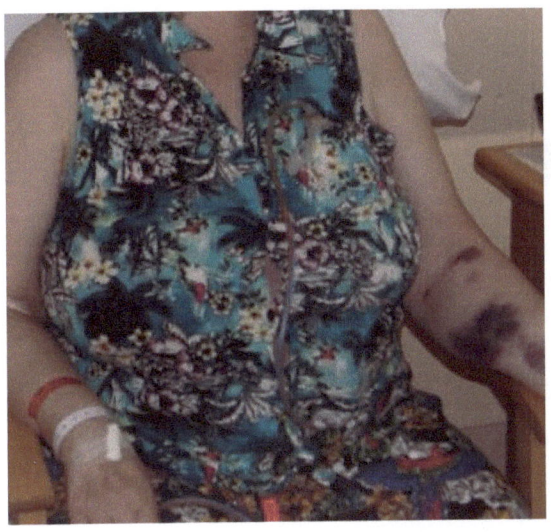

So that was me the day after the operation. I had to wear compression socks - which fitted very snugly - and an abdominal binder.

It was at this point I began getting some swelling around the midriff. This continued.

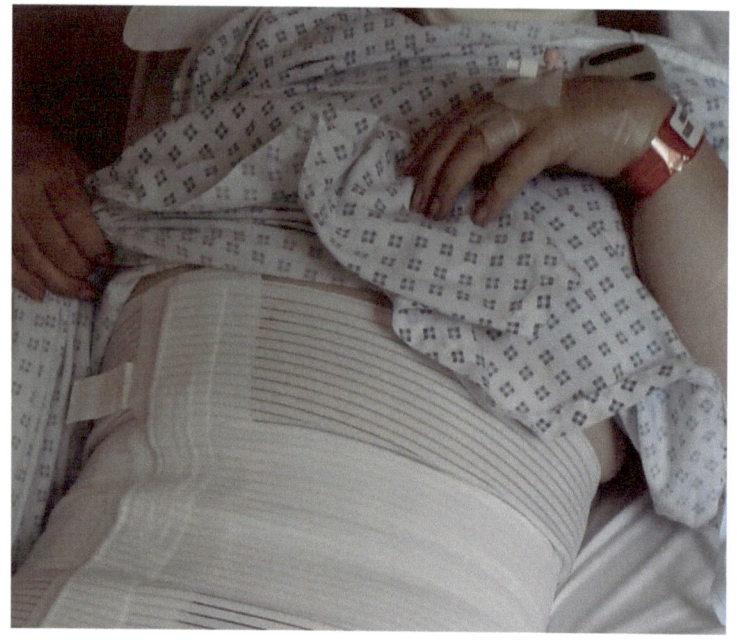

I developed breathing problems and bilateral pneumonia and was put on oxygen. I don't remember much about this at all.

You can see the development of the swelling now but what you can't see is how when they closed the diastasis it compressed my lungs and along with it came bilateral pneumonia.

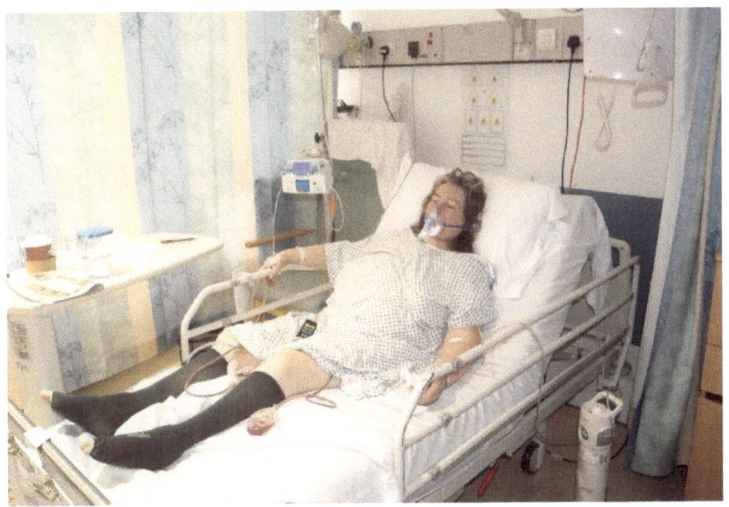

I was placed on:

- anti-coagulants
- two different types of antibiotics
- steroids
- two different types of inhalers
- pain medication

My SATS dropped rapidly during the night and I was rushed to another hospital which could deal with my breathing problems.

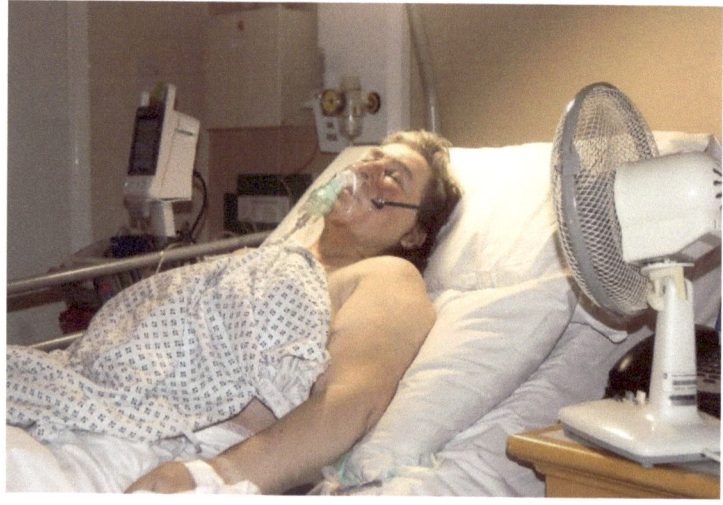

This picture of me above is just before I was taken to another hospital.

They had the fan going to try and reduce my rapidly mounting temperature.

I was placed on a drip as I was too weak to drink. I think this is when the pain hit me, too but as I was in hospital it was managed very well. It was very different when I eventually went home though because I did not have the same equipment at home to help me.

I didn't realise how much of a difference it would make.

Eventually, I was transferred back to the hospital where I'd had the operation. I had my own private room and it was a lot quieter.

The physiotherapist came to show me how to breathe properly as I still had the breathing problems and unfortunately, I continued to swell.

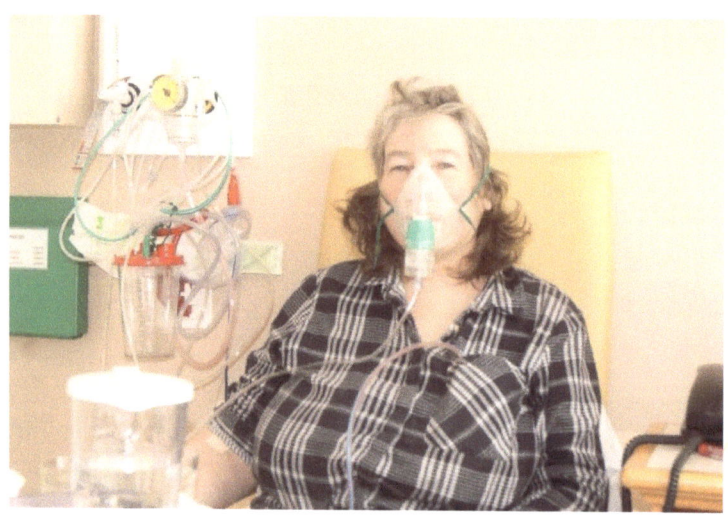

I had two abdominal drains in after surgery as well as a catheter. The abdominal drains did a good job of draining any fluid in the cavities which were formed when tissue was removed. This helps to avoid the development of seromas.

I grew to hate the abdominal drains which were attached to a metre length of tubing with a bulb on the end. When the bulb was full of fluid and blood, it had to be measured and a record kept.

One end of the tubing is stitched into your groin and, of course, the other end has the bulb attached. If they are pulled accidentally, there is a major 'ouch' factor. I found that it was easiest to transfer them to my pockets to carry them around initially, although when I needed to use the toilet it was a major performance juggling clothing. In the end it was easier buying a bigger bra and tucking them in there for the duration.

When I down to less than 25mls of fluid in the bulb daily, the drains were taken out. This is when further problems started.

Seromas are very common after major abdominal surgery. I wish I had been told this before the operation, but I wasn't.

The skin doesn't stick together very well after surgery and fluid forms in the space, in some people, until healing takes place.

I was one of those people who formed bags of fluid. Their official name is a seroma. When seromas form they need to be drained. This entails the surgeon sticking a needle into the space in the abdomen and withdrawing the fluid.

It isn't actually as painful as it sounds. The first seroma which was drained elicited 600mls of fluid which is quite a lot.

I think everyone was hoping that the tissues would stick together at that point but they didn't. I continued to develop seromas and these had to be drained another four times.

I was really getting quite weary at this point as I hadn't recovered from the pneumonia and I was having to trail backwards and forwards from the hospital to have things checked and be drained.

In the end the surgeon decided that he would need to insert another abdominal drain so six weeks after the first operation, I had another to insert another single drain on the right hand side. This was undertaken using local anaesthetic and took about an hour.

It was a number of weeks before I was hardly draining anything again and the abdominal drain could be removed. I don't really know why it had practically stopped draining before – when it was taken out – then started producing fluid which required another drain.

The drain was inserted in a slightly different place and once the tubing was removed the skin tethered.

So the picture below is taken 7 weeks after the operation and you can see that there is still considerable swelling.

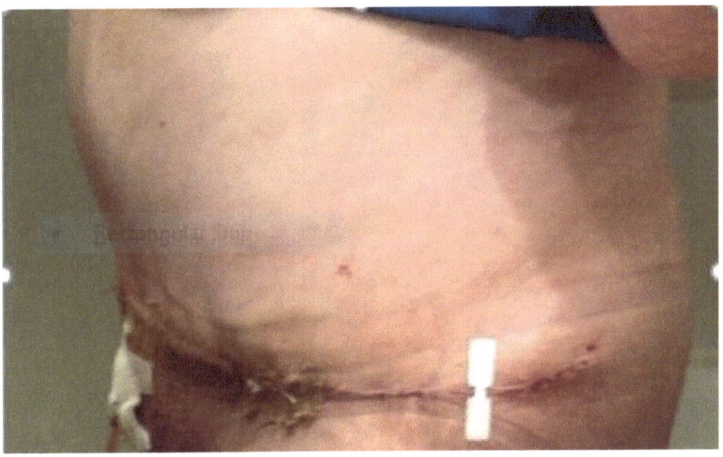

The scar is quite pronounced at this stage, too.

I wish that I could say that the difficulties stopped there but they didn't.

When an operation to close a diastasis rectus is performed the navel has to be separated from where it is attached in the abdomen. This has the potential for infections and, unfortunately. I had a number of infections which came on quite rapidly.

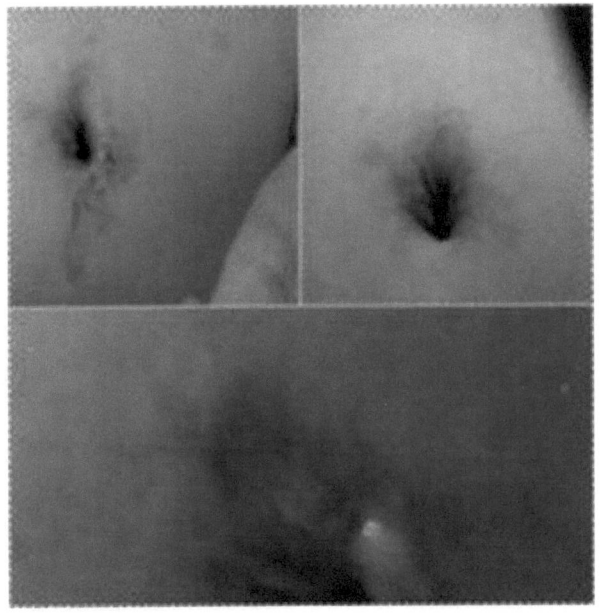

These were quickly cleared up by dropping chloramphenicol eye drops into the navel. They did re -occur quite frequently for the first year though.

I had to have a revision operation one year after but this, although it was undertaken under general anaesthetic was only a day case and I recovered fairly well.

Shortly after the first operation, the consultant asked me if I had indigestion as the operation often caused this. I didn't at the time of asking but have developed it since and have to take daily medication to control it.

I still have pain where the skin tethered where one of the abdominal drains was inserted. It is only minor but it needs mentioning as a possible complication. I have also developed lymphoedema in my legs which is another post-operative complication which I wasn't told about.

Lymphoedema is a long term condition which needs managing on a daily basis so these are all things which need to be considered before going ahead with an operation of this type.

There is no doubt that the huge 'bump' has gone and I am delighted about that since I was unable to find any clothes to fit me. On balance the operation was worth it just for that.

I am also able to stand for longer now without having to bend over and relieve the pain. This means I can go out shopping and stand in queues. I don't think people understand how debilitating this common condition is. Calling it mummy tummy makes it sound like something which is fairly innocuous but it does cause serious backache and is disabling. It can also cause constipation as well as self-esteem issues.

In spite of all the problems and with the benefit of hindsight, I would do it all again but I would have a better support structure in place for the first six weeks at least and I would also make sure that I had aids which would enable me to get into bed and also turn over. This was something that I could not do without my husband's help and I am a fairly stoic person.

I still have a fairly pronounced scar but it does not bother me since it cannot be seen as it is below the panty line. Maybe it will continue to fade. I don't know. It is now two and a half years since the first operation but it was a big operation when you consider the size of the abdominal gap.

Another bonus was that I used to get recurring sciatica for weeks on end. Since the operation this has disappeared so from that point of view the operation has saved me from years of future suffering. Anyone who has ever had sciatica will know what I mean.

The surgeon did say I would only be able to eat small amounts after everything was put back in place as there would be less room. As it is, this is not something I have noticed but then I have never eaten huge amounts.

I think that if I have anything further to add it is that I wish there had been more information of the potential post-operative complications so that I could have made a more informed decision but now, knowing what they are, I would still have gone ahead.

I can now wear what I like and am just as active as I was before the condition developed. For me, it was a win-win situation.

Thank you for purchasing this book. Every time a book is purchased, a donation is made to one of the charities I am currently supporting.
These can be found on my author's website.
See below.

Other Health Related Books by the Author

- The Reluctant Bowel
- A Weighty Issue
- Sleep, Perchance to Dream
- The Journey: EDS and chronic pain
- The MND diet: using nutrition to slow down the progress of neurodegeneration
- A Necessary Sorrow
- Treat infection Naturally
- Successful Aging
- Taking another Road: Pain: its causes and what can be done about it
- Osteoarthritis and Pain
- A Treatment Strategy for Migraine

These can be found here on the author's page

https://www.amazon.co.uk/-/e/B07BPQZ5CD

You may also be interested in the semi-autobiographical trilogy of the authors life found in these three books

- The Prejudged
- Where the Blackbird Never Sings
- A Summer's Symphony

And the author's children's books

- Fanny and Victorian Jack
- Fanny and the Gamekeeper's Cottage

www.ingramcontent.com/pod-product-compliance
Lightning Source LLC
Chambersburg PA
CBHW040351220526
45473CB00009B/2855